I0767021

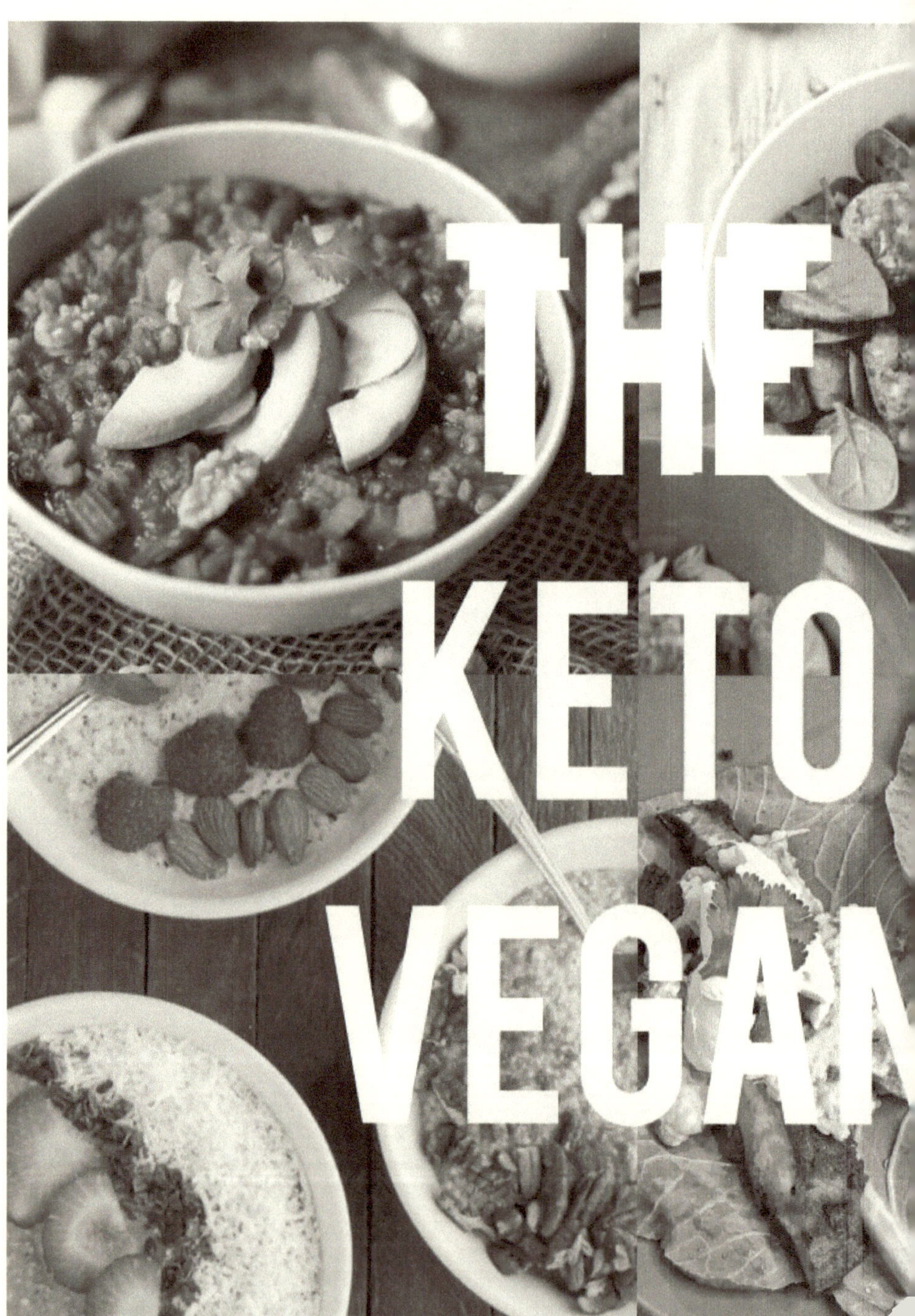
THE
KETO
VEGAN

TABLE OF CONTENTS

CHAPTER 3: THE KETO VEGAN

CHAPTER 1
THE "KETOGENIC" DIET

I'm sure by now you've probably heard the word "keto" come up many times in conversations about dieting with friends and colleagues, and I'm also sure most of you left the conversation still scratching your head. So just what is this keto diet? The ketogenic diet is a very low-carb, high-fat diet that shares many similarities with the Atkins and low-carb diets. It involves drastically reducing carbohydrate intake to between 20g and 100g per day and replacing it with fat. This reduction in carbs puts your body into a metabolic state called ketosis.

Ketosis is a metabolic state characterized by raised levels of ketone bodies in the body tissues, which is typically pathological in conditions such as diabetes, or may be the consequence of a diet that is very low in carbohydrates.

How can putting your body into ketosis benefit you? According to thrivestrive.com, one of the pros of ketosis is the weight loss. When the body slips into ketosis, it burns stored body fat for energy leaving you feeling fuller on less calories. There are claims that being in ketosis lowers blood pressure, which in turn makes your heart healthier. Ketosis helps fight type 2 diabetes by maintaining blood sugar levels, which in turn will help you focus better. Ketosis occurs when people eat a low- or no-carb diet and molecules called ketones build up in their bloodstream.

How can putting your body into ketosis negatively affect you? "Keto diets should only be used under clinical supervision and only for brief periods," Francine Blinten, R.D. "Anyone with type 2 diabetes can benefit from weight loss and a reduced-carb diet because it will improve insulin sensitivity". The most common negative side effect is something called the "Keto Flu" where you may experience the following:

- Headache.
- Fatigue.
- Brain fog.

- Increased hunger
- Poor sleep
- Nausea
- Decreased physical performance

The keto flu typically lasts a week and generally a not fun experience. But is there a way to pacify these symptoms? Absolutely, one way is by getting in essential mineral like these:

1. Calcium
2. Chloride
3. Magnesium
4. Phosphorus
5. Potassium
6. Sodium

Another way to deal with symptoms is by increasing your salt, water, and fat intake. Whenever you are feeling symptoms of the keto flu, take a teaspoon of table salt and chug a quarter gallon of water. If symptoms persist, I suggest increasing your carb count and see how you feel after that, but if you still feel sick it might be time to throw in the towel.

Another common side effect of the keto diet is enhanced body odor and bad breath called "keto breath". These side effects have been reported by meat and dairy eating individuals, in my opinion the side effects are due to high consumption of meat, dairy and other highly acidic products. Our bodies are over 70% water and naturally alkaline, when we introduce foods that are highly acidic it throws our bodies off balance.

EXAMPLE KETO GROCERY LIST (as a meat-eater)

- Alfalfa sprouts
- Almonds
- Artichoke hearts
- Arugula
- Arugula
- Asparagus
- Avocado
- Beans, green, snap, string
- Beef, preferably fattier cuts like steak, veal, roast, and ground beef
- Bell peppers
- Blackberries
- Blue cheese
- Blueberries
- Bok choy
- Bok choy (pak choi)
- Boston/bibb lettuce
- Brazil nuts
- Brie
- Broccoli florets

- Brussel sprouts
- Cabbage, green, red
- cashews
- Cauliflower
- Cauliflower florets
- Celery
- Celery
- Cheddar or Colby jack
- Cherries, sour, fresh, w/o pit
- Chia seeds
- Chicory greens
- Chinese cabbage (pak-choi)
- Chives
- Choose the highest-quality meat and eggs you can afford
- Collard greens
- Cottage cheese (2% fat)
- Cottage cheese (creamed)
- Cranberries, raw
- Cream cheese
- Cucumber (with peel)
- Cucumbers
- Currants, fresh, red and white
- Daikon radish
- Eggplant
- Eggs, including deviled, fried, scrambled and boiled — use the whole egg
- Endive
- Escarole
- Fennel, bulb

- Feta
- Flaxseeds
- Goat cheese
- Goat meat
- Gooseberries
- Gouda
- Grass-fed and organic red meats
- grass-fed butter
- Green and white cabbage
- Greens
- Ground fish, including mackerel, tuna, salmon, trout, halibut, cod, catfish and mahi-mahi
- Hazelnuts
- heavy cream
- Heavy whipping cream or double cream (fluid)
- Heavy whipping cream or double cream (whipped)
- High fat dairy like ghee
- Iceberg lettuce
- Jicama
- Lamb meat
- Lard
- Lettuce
- Loganberries
- Loose-leaf lettuce
- Macadamia nuts
- Melon
- Mozzarella (whole milk)
- Mung bean sprouts

- Mushrooms, button
- Mustard (Dijon)
- Mustard (yellow)
- Okra
- Olives, black
- Olives, green
- Onion
- Organ meats, including heart, liver, tongue, kidney and offal
- Parmesan
- Parsley
- Pecans
- Peppers, green bell
- Peppers, red bell
- Pesto sauce
- Pickapeppa sauce
- Pickle (dill or kosher)
- Pimento or roasted red pepper
- Pine nuts
- pistachios
- Pork, including pork loin, tenderloin, chops, ham, bacon
- Poultry, including chicken, quail, duck, turkey and wild game — try to focus on the   darker, fattier meats
- Pumpkin seeds
- Radicchio
- Radishes
- Raspberries
- Ricotta (whole milk)
- Romaine lettuce

- Salsa, green (no added sugar)
- Salsa, red
- Scallion/green onion
- Serrano chili pepper
- Sesame seeds
- Shellfish, including oysters, clams, crab, mussels and lobster
- Sour cream
- Soy sauce
- Spinach
- Sriracha
- Strawberries
- Sunflower seeds and sunflower seed butter
- Swiss
- Tabasco or other hot sauce
- Taco sauce
- Tahini (sesame paste)
- Tahini (sesame seed paste)
- Tomato, cherry
- Vinegar, balsamic
- Walnuts
- Wasabi paste
- Watercress
- Worcestershire sauce
- Yogurt (plain unsweetened/whole milk)
- Zucchini

When choosing your meats and seafood, it's important to consider the source. While it can be tempting to find conventionally raised meat on sale, you'll be doing your health a huge disservice. See, conventional meats are jacked up with hormones to make the animals grow bigger and faster so they'll be more profitable in the end. But these hormones — such as the stress one cortisol — don't just disappear when your meat is cooked. These are transferred to your system and can wreak havoc on your body when you eat them. To avoid this, it pays to spend the extra cash on grass-fed meats and organic options.

When following a ketogenic diet, you want to get the majority of your carbohydrates from vegetables such as leafy greens, asparagus, broccoli, cauliflower and most other vegetables that grow above ground. Avoid starchy vegetables like potatoes, corn and parsnips. The rest of your carbohydrate intake should come from the carbs in nuts and seeds, the small amount in dairy and on occasion, from fruits like berries.

FOODS TO AVOID ON THE KETO DIET:

- Bread, pasta, rice, potatoes (including sweet potatoes), French fries, potato chips, porridge, muesli and so on. Avoid wholegrain products as well. Legumes, such as beans and lentils, are high in carbs too.

- o Just because you're following a high-fat ketogenic diet doesn't mean you should indulge in every fat you come across. All fats are not created equal.
- Grains: All wheat (bread, pasta, cereal, etc.), oats, rice, quinoa, barley
- Low-fat, reduced fat, and fat free milk
- Evaporated or condensed milk
  - o Once the fat has been removed in milk, sugar is added to fill in the gaps and make the milk taste better. It's this added sugar that will prevent you from reaching ketosis
- Half and half
  - o Don't go for this half milk/half cream mixture either. You're still getting a dose of sugar and less fat, two things that won't help you on keto
- Any form of cane sugar
- Honey (use one of these four low carb honey substitutes if you miss the taste or need the consistency in a recipe)
- Maple syrup
- High-fructose corn syrup
- Date syrup
- Agave syrup

<u>**Steer clear of these unhealthy fats:**</u>

#1: Hydrogenated and partially hydrogenated oils. These trans fats are found in packaged foods. They increase inflammation and your risk of developing heart disease, cancer, and high cholesterol.

> ➢ If you're relying on packaged foods to get you through keto, check the label and ditch any foods with these.

#2: Highly processed vegetable oils. Corn oil, peanut oil, canola oil, soybean oil, sunflower, and grapeseed oil are all fats that sound healthier than they actually are.

SAMPLE DAY OF MEALS ON KETO DIET (meat-eater)

BREAKFAST	LUNCH	DINNER
• 2 whole eggs	• 4 oz Salmon	• 4 oz grilled chicken
• 3 egg whites	• 1 cup Broccoli	• 3 cups raw spinach
• 2 slices	• 4 oz	• 2

turkey bacon • 1 avocado • 2 oz raw almonds	asparagus	tablespoons olive oil

CHAPTER 2
PLANT-BASED OR VEGAN DIET

What does it mean to be vegan? What is a plant-based diet? Are they the same thing? Veganism is the practice of abstaining from the use of animal products, particularly in diet, and an associated philosophy that rejects the commodity status of animals. A follower of the diet or the philosophy is known as a vegan. A plant-based diet is a diet based on foods derived from plants, including vegetables, whole grains, nuts, seeds, legumes and fruits, but with few or no animal products but you do not necessarily have to subscribe to the vegan philosophy. There is a difference, small but yes slightly different.

Eating a vegan or plant-based diet has a wide variety of benefits; however today I will only touch a few of those. By cutting animal fat and animal protein from your diet, the risk of diabetes, rheumatoid arthritis, hypertension, heart disease, various cancers and many health issues can be greatly reduced.

The vegan diet consists of far higher volumes of legumes, fruits, and vegetables, fiber, and vitamin C than most diets. These are believed to protect against a variety of cancers. Meat eaters are at a higher risk of colorectal and prostate cancers.

People on a vegan diet often take in fewer calories than a those on a standard Western diet, which leads me to the next benefit. You can expect stubborn body fat to melt away. A lower BMI is linked to lower overall concentrations of LDL cholesterol and slightly lower blood pressure, even compared with vegetarians who continue to drink animal milk.

Lower levels of harmful cholesterol mean that vegans have a lower risk of mortality from stroke and ischemic heart disease than people who eat meat.

EXAMPLE VEGAN GROCERY LIST:
- Anise
- Artichoke
- Azuki Beans
- Agave Syrup
- Alfalfa Sprouts
- Almond Butter
- Almond Milk
- Almond Yogurt
- Almonds
- Amaranth
- Apple Sauce
- Apples
- Apricots
- Arugula
- Arugula
- Asparagus
- Avocado
- Avocado
- Baby Spinach
- Baked Beans
- Baking Powder

- Bamboo Shoots
- Bananas
- Barley
- Basil
- Bay Leaf
- Bean Sprouts
- Beans
- Beet
- Bell Peppers
- Black Beans
- Black Eyed Peas
- Blackberries
- Blueberries
- Bok Choy
- Brazil Nuts
- Broccoli
- Broccoli
- Brown Rice
- Brussels Sprouts
- Buckwheat
- Bulgur
- Cabbage
- Canned Tomatoes
- Cannelini Beans
- Cantaloupe
- Carrots
- Cashew Butter
- Cashew Milk
- Cashews

- Cauliflower
- Celery
- Celery Seed
- Chamomile
- Chard
- Cheddar Style Shreds
- Cheese Slices
- Cherries
- Cherry Tomatoes
- Chestnuts
- Chia seeds
- Chia Seeds
- Chickpeas
- Chili powder
- Chilies
- Chives
- Chocolate Flavored Almond/Soy Milk
- Cilantro
- Clementines
- Clove
- Cocoa
- Coconut
- Coconut Milk
- Coconut Milk
- Coconut Milk Creamer
- Coconut Sugar
- Coconut Yogurt
- Coffee
- Coffee

- Collard
- Coriander
- Corn
- Corn
- Corn, Cornflakes
- Cornstarch
- Couscous
- Cream Cheese (non-dairy/plant based)
- Cucumber
- Cucumber
- Cumin
- Currants
- Curry
- Curry Paste
- Date Syrup
- Dill
- Durian
- Earth Balance Butter
- Edamame
- Eggplant
- Einkorn
- Endive
- Farro
- Fava Beans
- Fennel
- Figs
- Flax Milk
- Flax Seeds
- Garlic

- Garlic Powder
- Ginger
- Grapefruit
- Grapes
- Green Beans
- Green Onions
- Guacamole
- Guava
- Harissa
- Hazelnuts
- Hemp Milk
- Hemp Seeds
- Honeydew
- Hummus
- Ice Cream (Almond/Soy)
- Italian Seasoning
- Jackfruit
- Jalapeno Peppers
- Kale
- Kamut
- Kidney Beans
- Kiwis
- Kohlrabi
- Kumquats
- Lamb's Lettuce
- Leafy greens
- Leek
- Legumes
- Lemon Juice

- Lemongrass
- Lemons
- Lentils
- Lentils
- Lentils
- Lettuce
- Lima Beans
- Limes
- Lychees
- Macadamia Nuts
- Macadamia Nut Butter
- Mangoes
- Mangosteen
- Maple Syrup
- Marjoram
- Millet
- Miso Paste
- Mixed Salad
- Molasses
- Mozzarella Style Shreds (non-dairy/plant based)
- Mung Beans
- Mushrooms
- Mustard
- Navy Beans
- Nectarines
- Nutmeg
- Nutritional Yeast
- Oat Milk

- Oats
- Okra
- Olives
- Olives
- Onion Powder
- Onions
- Oranges
- Oregano
- Organic Cane Sugar
- Papayas
- Paprika
- Parsley
- Parsnip
- Passionfruit
- Pasta
- Peaches
- Peanut Butter
- Peas
- Peas
- Pecans
- Pepper
- Peppermint
- Persimmon
- Physalis
- Pine Nuts
- Pinto Beans
- Pistachios
- Plantains
- Plums

- Pomegranate
- Poppy Seed
- Potatoes
- Pumpkin
- Pumpkin Seeds
- Quinoa
- Radishes
- Raspberries
- Red Beans
- Red Pepper Flakes
- Rhubarb
- Rice Cakes
- Rice Milk
- Romaine Lettuce
- Rosemary
- Rye
- Saffron
- Salsa
- Salt
- Seitan
- Sesame Seeds
- Spelt
- Shallots
- Snow Peas
- Sour Cream (non-dairy/plant based)
- Sorrel
- Soy Beans
- Soy Milk
- Soy Milk Creamer

- Soy Products (Soy Beans, Tempeh, Tofu, Sauce)
- Soy Yogurt
- Spinach
- Split Peas
- Spring Greens
- Sprouts
- Squash
- Stevia
- Strawberries
- Sugar Snap Peas
- Sun Dried Tomatoes
- Sunflower Seeds
- Sunflower Seed Butter
- Sweet Potatoes
- Tahini
- Tea
- Tempeh (spiced/plain)
- Thyme
- Tofu (firm/soft/spiced)
- Tomatoes
- Tomatoes
- Tortillas
- Trail Mix
- Turmeric
- Turnip
- Turnip Tops
- Vanilla

- Vinegar (Apple Cider, Balsamic, Rice etc.)
- Walnuts
- Watercress
- Watermelon
- Wheat
- Wheatgrass
- White Beans
- White Bread
- White Rice
- Whole Grain Bread/Rolls
- Whole Grain Flour
- Whole Grain Pasta
- Wild Rice
- Yams
- Zucchini

FOODS TO AVOID ON A VEGAN DIET:
AVOID any animal products such as meat, fish, and dairy, and foods that contain animal products. Preferably you want to AVOID processed and artificial foods. Always check ingredient labels of all products you come across which will indicate when there may be "MILK, EGGS, SHELLFISH" in the product.

Tip : Downloading an app to scan food package bar codes for additional confirmation of no animal based ingredients within the product is a very helpful tool.

(Search "Is it Vegan?" in your app store which is a great app for this)

SAMPLE DAY OF MEALS EATING PLANT BASED / VEGAN:

Breakfast : <u>SCRAMBLE, SWEET POTATOES, & SAUSAGE</u>

- 4 oz extra firm tofu (crumble, season (salt, pepper, turmeric, nutritional yeast, garlic) sauté
- ½ cup sweet Potato (baked or boiled)
- Tofurky - Italian Sausage, sliced (1/2 sausage)
- Mushrooms - Grilled, ¼ cup

Steps:Combine tofu, spinach, tofurky sausage and mushrooms on frying pan. Stir-fry style with your favorite seasonings on medium,/high heat like an "egg and veggie scramble" . Bake or Boil sweet potato and sprinkle cinnamon and coconut sugar for added flavor

OR opt for a "sweet" option instead of "savory"

<u>Peanut Butter and Fruit Protein OAT BOWL</u>

- Oatmeal (Dry), 40 g
- Chia Seed, 1 tbsp
- Peanut Butter, 2 tbsp
- Hemp Seeds, 3 tbsp
- Banana, 1 medium 130g
- Giant - Strawberries, 1 cup

- Blueberries, 1 cup

Steps: Cooks oats with plant milk or water and add topping as desired

Dinner: <u>CHICKPEA & QUINOA TACOS</u>

- 2 fajita style tortillas
- Cooked Quinoa, 1 cup
- Canned Chickpeas (or boil raw chickpeas), 1 cup
- Sliced bell peppers sautéed
- Shredded Roasted Cabbage, 0.5 cup cooked
- Organic Shredded Carrots, 0.5 cup (85g)

Steps: Combine ingredients and cook as desired, add sesame oil, scallions, garlic and a drizzle of soy sauce to the quinoa & chickpeas for an asian style "fried rice" filling. Stack everything along with your shredded veggies into your tacos to make some yummy tacos. Drizzle on your favorite non-dairy/vegan sauce and fresh cilantro and diced tomatoes to top it off

CHAPTER 3
THE KETO VEGAN

By this chapter you should have a
general understanding of what it means to be a

keto dieter, and what it means to be a vegan or plant-based dieter. But what does it mean to be a keto vegan? Essentially, this would mean that you would follow both vegan and keto philosophies simultaneously. So, in a nutshell you will eat your fill of plant-based foods, primarily leafy greens, nuts, and soy-based meat replacements while keeping your total daily carb intake under 100 grams.

How can you benefit from eating this way? In my professional opinion, I would not suggest maintaining this way of eating longer than 30 days at a time. Running so low on carbs for so long isn't healthy. The keto philosophy requires you exclude a lot of fibrous, anti-cancerous, anti-oxidant rich foods. If you need to drop a couple of pounds for a wedding or a vacation I highly suggest this method over crash dieting and even traditional keto.

EXAMPLE KETO VEGAN GROCERY LIST

Be mindful of the carbohydrate/sugar content of some items listed below depending on the amount you consume.

- Almond Butter
- Artichokes
- Arugula
- Asparagus

- Avocados
- Baby bok choy
- Beet Greens
- Bell Peppers
- Broccoli
- Brussel Sprouts
- Cabbage
- Cashew Cheese
- Cauliflower
- Celery
- Chia Seeds
- Coconut Yogurt
- Collard Greens
- Cucumbers
- Dandelion Greens
- Edamame
- Eggplant
- Fennel
- Flaxseed Oil
- Green Beans
- Guacamole
- Hazelnut Butter
- Hearts of Palm
- Hemp Seeds
- Kale
- Kelp flakes
- Kelp noodles
- Lemons
- Limes

- Macadamia Nut Butter
- MCT Oil
- Mushrooms
- Mustard Greens
- Nori Sheets
- Nutritional Yeast
- Okra
- Olive Oil
- Onions
- Peanut Butter (natural/raw)
- Peppers
- Pumpkin Seeds
- Radishes
- Roasted Seaweed
- Shiritaki noodles
- Spinach
- Sunflower Seeds
- Swiss Chard
- Tempeh
- Tofu
- Tomatoes
- Turnips
- Watercress
- Zucchini

Fat: Coconut oil, coconut cream/milk, avocado, plant-based oils, nuts and seeds

Healthy protein: nut-based yogurts, soy proteins and high-protein veggies

Carbohydrates: Tomatoes, broccoli, onion, kale, spinach, brussels sprouts and raspberries

Some helpful Tips

- Cauliflower can be grated into "rice," or boiled and mashed like potatoes. You can slice zucchini into noodles to (sort of) replicate pasta.
- One of the best low-carb vegan proteins have been found to be hemp seeds, which provide 30g protein and 8g fiber which are not counted as carbs - in a half cup serving.

WHAT NOT TO EAT AS A KETO VEGAN:

- **High-carb fruits**
  - *Examples: Bananas, clementines, apples, kiwis and blueberries*
- **All grains**
  - Examples : Whole wheat breads, quinoa, oats and corn
- **Processed, natural and artificial sugars**

o *Examples: White sugar, cane sugar, agave, honey, maple syrup, Equal and Splenda*

- **Tubers**
  - o *Examples: Potatoes, taro and yams*

SAMPLE DAY OF MEALS AS A KETO VEGAN:

<table>
<tr><td>

Breakfast : <u>KETO BREAKFAST SCRAMBLE</u>
- 6 oz extra firm tofu (crumble, season (salt, pepper, turmeric, nutritional yeast, garlic) sauté
- 2 cups mushrooms (grilled)
- 2 cups raw spinach
- 1tbsp coconut oil
- Fresh black berries or blueberries on the side

Steps:Combine tofu, spinach, tofurky sausage and mushrooms on frying pan. Stir-fry style with your favorite seasonings on medium,/high heat like an "egg and veggie scramble"

</td></tr>
<tr><td>

Lunch : <u>AVOCADO KALE SALAD</u>
- 3 cups chopped raw kale
- 3oz raw almonds

--Dressing—
- 2 tbsp olive oil
- 2 tbsp fresh lemon juice
- 1 tbsp nutritional yeast
- ½ hass avocado
- ½ tsp garlic powder
- ¼ tsp onion powder

</td></tr>
</table>

- ¼ tsp pepper
- 2 tsp pink salt/sea salt

Steps:Combine dressing ingredients and massage into kale, top with whole or sliced almonds

Dinner : <u>ZOODLES</u>

- 1 medium or large zucchini (spiralized)
- 1 cup canned tomatoes
- 2 tbsp olive oil
- 1 tbsp nutritional yeast
- ½ cup sliced mushrooms
- 6oz crumbled tofu

Steps: Stew ingredients together (aside from the zoodles) add salt herbs and spices to taste (fresh basil, parsley) and lay over lightly sautéed zucchini or keep them raw. Garnish with fresh basil or parsley. Enjoy

Snack : <u>CHIA SEED PUDDING</u> (pre-make <u>pudding night before)</u>

- 2 tablespoons chia seeds
- 1 cup coconut or almond milk (unsweetened)
- vanilla stevia drops or preferred sweetener, to taste
  - Mix chia seeds with your chosen milk, cover and refrigerate overnight.
  - Add more liquid as needed to reach desired consistency (optional). Sweeten to taste and serve with toppings of choice.

Toppings suggestions: add fresh blueberries, almonds , unsweetened coconut flakes. Drizzle fresh almond butter on top for an added touch of yummyness